DIABETES GUIDE TO

Enjoying Foods of the World

CONSTANCE BROWN-RIGGS
MSEd, RDN, CDE, CDN

JESSICA JONES
MS, RDN, CDE

Academy of Nutrition and Dietetics
Chicago, IL

eat® right. Academy of Nutrition and Dietetics

Academy of Nutrition and Dietetics
120 S. Riverside Plaza, Suite 2190
Chicago, IL 60606

Diabetes Guide to Enjoying Foods of the World

ISBN 978-0-88091-950-0
Catalog Number 950017

The views expressed in this publication are those of the authors and do not necessarily reflect policies and/or official positions of the Academy of Nutrition and Dietetics. Mention of product names in this publication does not constitute endorsement by the authors or the Academy of Nutrition and Dietetics. The Academy of Nutrition and Dietetics disclaims responsibility for the application of the information contained herein.

Calorie and carbohydrate data are approximate amounts, derived primarily from the US Department of Agriculture, Agricultural Research Service, Nutrient Data Laboratory. USDA National Nutrient Database for Standard Reference, Release 28, 2016; ndb.nal.usda.gov/ndb, and the USDA Food and Nutrient Database for Dietary Studies (FNDDS); https://reedir.arsnet.usda.gov/codesearchwebapp. Other online databases were consulted for food items not found in the USDA database.

10 9 8 7 6 5 4 3 2 1

For more information on the Academy of Nutrition and Dietetics, visit www.eatright.org.

Contents

About the Authors

Constance Brown-Riggs, MSEd, RDN, CDE, CDN, is an award winning registered dietitian, certified diabetes educator, and past national spokesperson for the Academy of Nutrition and Dietetics. She is the author of the *African American Guide to Living Well with Diabetes* and *Eating Soulfully and Healthyly with Diabetes*. Connie specializes in nutrition, diabetes, and cultural issues that impact the health and healthcare of people of color. Connie's ability to translate her extensive academic and clinical knowledge of medical nutrition into clear, understandable terms has made her a nationally respected and much sought-after speaker, educator, and author. Her work has appeared in books for health professionals and health-conscious consumers, and she has been a featured expert in national magazines such as *Essence, Real Health*, and *Diabetic Cooking*.

Jessica Jones, MS, RDN, CDE, is a registered dietitian nutritionist and certified diabetes educator with a focus on intuitive eating. Currently, she provides outpatient nutrition counseling in weight management, prediabetes/diabetes, heart disease, gastrointestinal issues, and plant-based eating at University of California, San Francisco. Using her bachelor of arts in journalism and master of science in nutrition, Jessica has penned hundreds of articles about food, health, and culture for publications like SELF.com, Buzzfeed, and *Today's Dietitian*. In 2017, Jessica released her first cookbook, *28-Day Plant-Powered Health Reboot*. She is the cofounder of the website Food Heaven Made Easy, a one-stop-shop for delicious and nutritious living. Jones also cohosts *The Food Heaven Podcast*, which delivers practical, evidenced-based nutrition education that listeners can trust.

Introduction

Having diabetes doesn't prevent you from living a rich, healthy life, and it also doesn't mean you won't be able to enjoy the authentic ethnic foods you've grown up with or that you're interested in trying. If you eat wisely and well, you can still enjoy all the flavors of the world, despite your diabetes. That's exactly why the *Diabetes Guide to Enjoying Foods of the World* was created—to show you how!

Every cuisine has its own native foods and preparation methods that can enhance its healthy aspects. Of course, every cuisine also features some foods and preparation methods that could derail a healthy diet. For each of the many different cuisines covered in the *Diabetes Guide to Enjoying Foods of the World,* you'll find the headings Healthy Pleasures and Dishes Reserved for Special Occasions (or Smaller Portions) that clearly identify healthy dishes (and dishes reserved for special occasions) for those on a healthy diet. The Healthy Pleasures options fit well in any sensible diet, and the Dishes Reserved for Special Occasions have higher levels of solid fats, sugars, starches, or sodium. At the end of each chapter, you'll find calorie and carbohydrate ("carbs") data for common foods from the cuisine to help you make and follow a meal plan.

Regardless of the meal planning strategy you follow and whether you are eating at home or away from home, the basic principles of healthy eating are the same:

- Limit foods that are high in sugar.
- Eat smaller portions spread out over the day.

- Be careful about when and how many carbohydrates you eat.
- Eat a variety of whole-grain foods, fruits, and vegetables every day.
- Eat less fat.
- Limit your intake of alcohol.
- Use less salt.

Diabetes Nutrition Guidelines

The Diabetes Nutrition Guidelines from the American Diabetes Association (ADA) state that the principles of a healthy diet are the same for people with diabetes as they are for everyone else. The ADA recommends that adults diagnosed with diabetes should consume a healthy diet focused on nutrient-dense foods, such as vegetables, fruits, whole grains, nonfat or low-fat milk and milk products, lean meats and poultry, fish and seafood, eggs, beans, peas, nuts, and seeds. They also recommend that these foods should be prepared without added solid fats, sugars, starches, and sodium.

The guidelines emphasize that there is no "one-size-fits-all" or "right" way for a person with diabetes to eat. Instead, the ADA recommend that people with diabetes follow a sensible diet based on their individual preferences, cultures, religious beliefs, traditions, and diabetes management goals.

It's certainly true there is no single perfect diabetes diet, but there are meal planning tools and strategies that can help you choose foods wisely and thus help you manage your diabetes. Carbohydrate counting, the plate method of meal planning, and portion control are three of those strategies. Read about each of the strategies below, and then apply them to your favorite dishes from around the world.

Carbohydrate Counting

Carbohydrate counting, one of the most commonly used methods of diabetes meal planning today, gives you lots of flexibility in your food choices and helps you understand how different foods affect your blood glucose—also called blood sugar—level.

The more carbohydrate-containing foods you eat during a meal or snack, the more glucose will enter your bloodstream. Thus, keeping close track of how many carbohydrates you consume is the best way to determine just the right amount of carbohydrates needed to keep your blood glucose levels in your target range.

A list of carbohydrate goals per meal or snack is sometimes referred to as a *carbohydrate budget*. It's reasonable for most adults to consume 45 to 60 grams of carbohydrates at each meal and 15 to 30 grams at each snack. To determine the amount of carbohydrates that are right for you, track how many grams of carbohydrates you consume at any given meal or snack, and then check your blood glucose levels 2 hours later. If this method is not successful for you, consult a registered dietitian nutritionist (RDN) to help you determine the right amount of carbohydrates for your diet.

Plate Method of Meal Planning

The plate method of meal planning is an easy way to control your portions and carbohydrate intake. It requires no calculating, weighing, or measuring. The method is very simple: When you serve yourself a meal, make sure half of your plate is full of nonstarchy vegetables, such as broccoli, cauliflower, spinach, or asparagus. A quarter of your plate should be dedicated to starchy foods, like potatoes, pasta, bread, corn, or kidney beans, and the last quarter should be reserved for fish, poultry, meat, or a plant-based protein.

This method works particularly well when eating in restaurants and away from home. Covering half of your plate with nonstarchy vegetables will automatically reduce your carbohydrate count.

Sizing Up Portions

Many people are confused when it comes to portions and servings, and they often use the terms interchangeably. Yet portions and servings are two completely different measurements.

A *portion* is the amount of food you choose to eat; a *serving* is a unit of measure used to describe the recommended amount of food from each food group. The following chart will help you size your portions to maintain better control of your blood glucose levels.

A Serving of …   Looks Like …

Grain/Starch Products

1 cup cereal flakes	A small adult fist
1 pancake or 1 slice of bread	A stack of DVDs
½ cup cooked rice, pasta, potatoes, or beans	½ baseball
1 slice of cornbread	A small bar of soap

Vegetables and Fruits

1 cup salad greens	A small adult fist
½ cup cooked vegetables	½ baseball
1 baked potato	A small adult fist
1 medium fruit	A baseball
¼ cup raisins	A large egg

Dairy and Cheese

1½ oz cheese	Four stacked dice
½ cup ice cream	A small fist

Meat and Alternatives

3 oz meat, fish (thick cut), or poultry	A deck of cards
3 oz grilled or baked fish fillet	A checkbook
2 Tbsp peanut butter	A ping-pong ball

Fats

1 tsp margarine or butter-like spread	The tip of your thumb

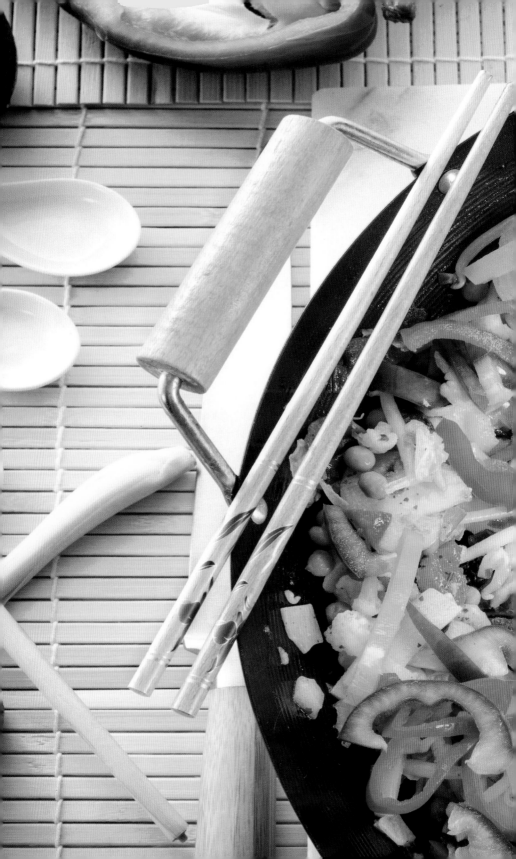

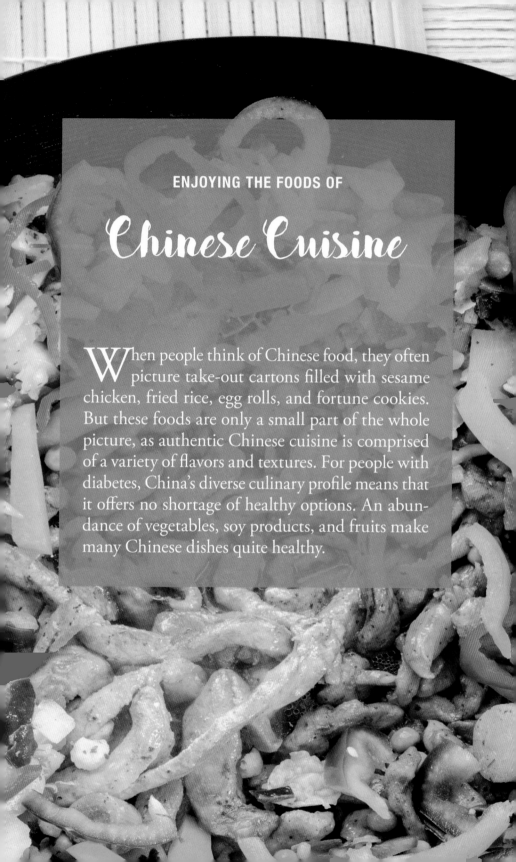

ENJOYING THE FOODS OF

Chinese Cuisine

When people think of Chinese food, they often picture take-out cartons filled with sesame chicken, fried rice, egg rolls, and fortune cookies. But these foods are only a small part of the whole picture, as authentic Chinese cuisine is comprised of a variety of flavors and textures. For people with diabetes, China's diverse culinary profile means that it offers no shortage of healthy options. An abundance of vegetables, soy products, and fruits make many Chinese dishes quite healthy.

Strategies for Healthy Eating

Choose lean proteins. Choose dishes that use tofu, also known as soybean curd, in lieu of meat, as tofu is low in saturated fat and high in protein. Roasted pork, chicken, and fish are also great lean sources of animal protein. When dining out, make sure to order meats that are roasted, steamed, or stir fried with small amounts of oil. Steer clear of any meats described as fried, batter fried, or crispy.

Focus on vegetables. Always choose mixed dishes that list vegetables in their descriptions, such as steamed chicken with broccoli or roasted pork with mixed vegetables, or try a vegetarian dish. Make sure to ask the server to add extra vegetables to your order, or order steamed vegetables on the side. Avoid vegetables that have been dipped in batter and fried because these preparations will increase the calorie and carbohydrate count.

Eat rice and noodles in moderation. Portion control is a must when it comes to rice—whether it's white or brown—and noodles. These are high-carbohydrate foods, and overconsumption of them can affect blood glucose levels. Diabetes experts recommended that half of your plate should be filled with nonstarchy vegetables, like Chinese broccoli, bean sprouts, or bok choy, and rice or noodles should be no more than a quarter of your plate. Fill the remaining quarter with a lean protein choice.

Be aware of added sodium and sugar. When preparing Chinese cuisine at home, limit the amount of sauce you use, and choose low-sodium types of soy and other sauces. To control the amount of sodium and sugar in your meal when dining out, be sure to specify that no monosodium glutamate (better known as MSG) is used, and be sure to request sauce on the side so you can control the amount you consume. Many Chinese restaurants provide low-sodium soy sauce as an option. Sugar and cornstarch are often added to Chinese sauces and marinades, such as *hoisin*, plum, and duck sauce.

Eat sweets in moderation. Opt for fresh fruit or a small serving of vanilla ice cream; each provides about 15 grams of carbohydrates. Steer clear of fried bananas due to the batter involved, as it increases the amount of carbohydrates. A better choice is a fortune cookie.

Healthy Pleasures

Chicken *chow mein* Chicken stir fried with a mixture of vegetables, like carrots, water chestnuts, mushrooms, and noodles

> **TIP** *Save on carbohydrates by asking for more vegetables and fewer noodles.*

Hot and sour soup A spicy soup made with red peppers and vinegar

Lo mein Parboiled Chinese egg noodles topped with a mixture of stir-fried vegetables, such as onions, snow peas, julienned carrots, and sliced button mushrooms; served plain or topped with marinated pork, shrimp, beef, or chicken

> **TIP** *Top with chicken or shrimp and ask for extra vegetables. Limit the noodle portion to a quarter of your plate.*

Steamed dumplings Small dumplings typically filled with onion and bamboo shoots and chicken, pork, or shrimp

> **TIP** *Steamed dumplings make a great low-carbohydrate appetizer*

Dishes Reserved for Special Occasions (or Smaller Portions)

Egg roll Deep-fried *wonton* wrapper stuffed with cabbage, carrots, bean sprouts, and other vegetables, as well as pork, shrimp, or chicken; high in fat and has more carbohydrates than the average slice of bread

Fried rice Steamed white rice stir fried in soy sauce and sesame oil with onions, peas, diced carrots, fried eggs, baby corn, and sometimes meat (chicken, beef, or pork); high in fat, carbohydrates, and sodium

Moo shu **pork** Sliced or shredded pork marinated in *hoisin* sauce and stir fried in sesame or peanut oil; low in carbohydrates but high in fat and sodium

Pot sticker Small steamed and fried dough pastries filled with meat (pork, chicken, or beef), cabbage, scallions, and ginger; high in fat, carbohydrates, and sodium

Sesame chicken battered, deep-fried, and glazed boneless chicken breast or thigh cooked in a sweet sauce and served with steamed broccoli or another vegetable; very high in fat, carbohydrates, and sodium

Sweet and sour chicken Small cubes of white-meat chicken battered, deep-fried, and coated with a sweet and sour sauce; high in fat and carbohydrates

Chinese Cuisine
Nutrition Facts

Food	Serving Size	Calories	Carbs (grams)
Chicken *chow mein*, no noodles	1 cup	185	9
Duck sauce	1 Tbsp	81	20
Egg roll (beef or pork)	1 roll (2-3 oz)	177	18
Fortune cookie	1 cookie	30	7
Fried rice (vegetable)	1 cup	238	45
Hoisin sauce	1 Tbsp	35	7
Hot and sour soup	1 cup	91	10
Lo mein (vegetable)	1 cup	165	27
Moo shu pork	1 cup	228	6
Plum sauce	1 Tbsp	35	8
Pot stickers (pork and vegetable)	3 pieces (3 oz)	118	12
Sesame chicken	1 cup	738	68
Steamed dumplings filled with meat, poultry, or seafood	4 medium dumplings (5 oz)	167	16
Sweet and sour chicken	3 pieces (2 oz)	138	13

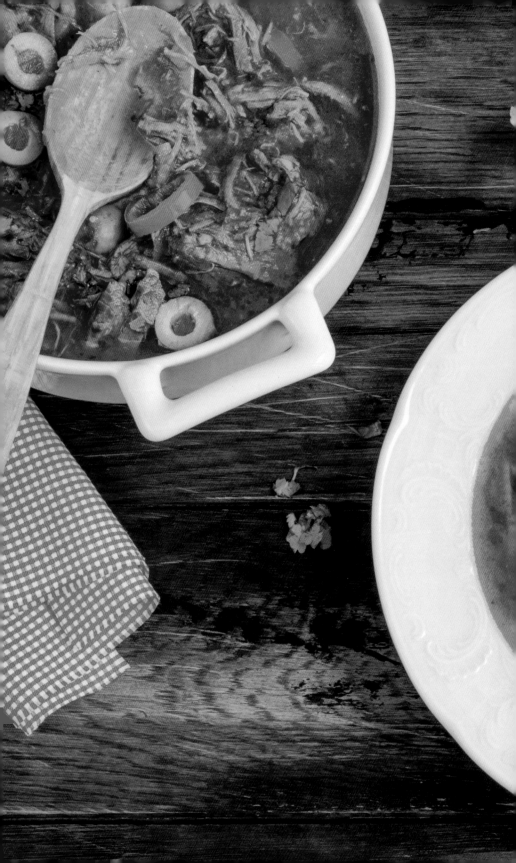

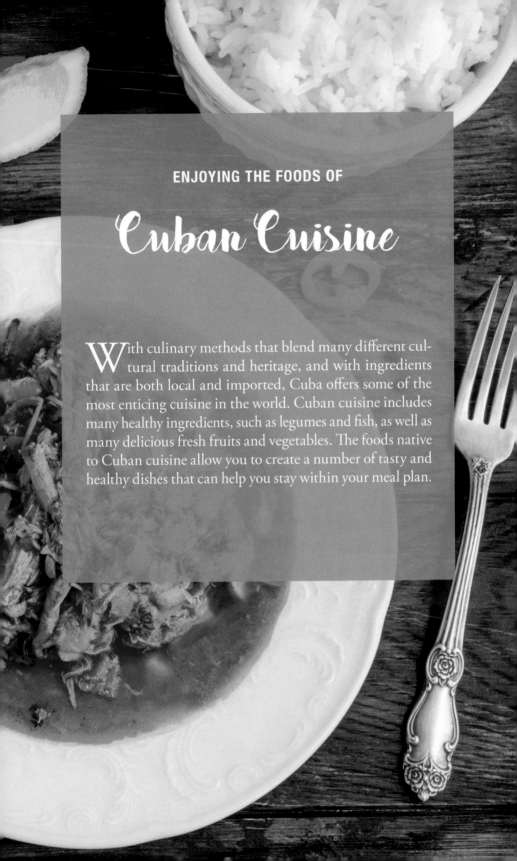

ENGOYING THE FOODS OF

Cuban Cuisine

With culinary methods that blend many different cultural traditions and heritage, and with ingredients that are both local and imported, Cuba offers some of the most enticing cuisine in the world. Cuban cuisine includes many healthy ingredients, such as legumes and fish, as well as many delicious fresh fruits and vegetables. The foods native to Cuban cuisine allow you to create a number of tasty and healthy dishes that can help you stay within your meal plan.

Strategies for Healthy Eating

Focus on legumes. Legume-containing dishes, including pigeon peas, lentils, black beans, and chickpeas, are popular throughout Cuba and offer many health advantages, such as being high in protein, low in fat, and high in fiber. A half cup of legumes has 15 grams of carbohydrates.

Enjoy fresh seafood. Fresh fish dishes, especially when poached, are a Healthy Pleasure. Fish provides a low-fat source of protein, and some types of fish are high in beneficial omega-3 fatty acids, which help protect the heart.

Eat fresh fruits and vegetables. Cuba has abundant fresh fruits and vegetables, such as avocados, bananas, *calabazas* (a type of tropical pumpkin), papayas, pineapples, and tomatoes. Fruits and vegetables are high in fiber, which helps you stay regulated and feel full.

Keep fat and sodium levels low. Many traditional Cuban dishes tend to be salty. Consuming too much sodium can lead to high blood pressure and can increase your risk of stroke and heart failure. Try to choose baked dishes, rather than fried, and stick to non–cured meats when possible, as they are lower in sodium.

Eat sweets in moderation. Sweets, including cakes, pastries, puddings, and cookies, are popular desserts and snacks in Cuba. Examples include *flan*, candied ripe plantains, and baked bananas. Choose fresh fruit for your sweet treats whenever possible, as the fiber in the fruit will slow the release of the natural fruit sugars into the bloodstream.

Healthy Pleasures

À la vizcaína Spanish-style salted codfish stew that includes potatoes, onions, garlic, and capers

> **TIP** *If you are making this at home, consider adding zucchini instead of potatoes or tossing in a bit of sautéed spinach for more fiber.*

Calabaza Usually referred to as Cuban squash; actually a cross between a squash and pumpkin; a good source of fiber and beta carotene

> **TIP** *If you're dining out and vegetables seem limited on the menu, ask for a side of steamed or boiled calabaza to increase the meal's fiber content. Any soups or stews made with calabaza are typically a healthy choice.*

Cocido de garbanzos Spanish-style stew made with chickpeas, cabbage, pork, and sausage that may also include onions, carrots, bell peppers, garlic, and olive oil

Cuban *tortilla* Usually contains eggs, potatoes, onions, garlic, and spices; the eggs become the "tortilla," similar to an American omelet; protein in the eggs balance the carbohydrates in the potatoes making it a good combination of nutrition and flavor

Ropa vieja Shredded beef often served on tortillas or over rice; contains beef, tomato paste, tomato sauce, onions, green bell peppers, garlic, olive oil, and spices

Sancocho Hearty stew that features many of Cuba's native root vegetables—squash, yuca, yams, or potatoes; often includes plantains, beans, lentils, or pigeon peas; most recipes include some type of meat, usually beef or pork

Dishes Reserved for Special Occasions (or Smaller Portions)

Arroz frito Cuban version of fried rice; can contain hidden sugars in the form of pineapple juice

Cuban bread Similar to French bread; small portions may be okay, but large portions will be high in carbohydrates

Cuban sandwich Sandwich made with ham, roasted pork, Swiss cheese, pickles, mustard, and sometimes salami; relatively high in sodium.

Flan Custard dessert with a layer of caramel on top; high in sugar and carbohydrates

Fried *tostones* Plantain slices pressed and fried in olive oil; fried makes it higher in fat and calories

Fried yuca Fried root vegetable also known as *cassava*; as with fried *tostones*, higher in fat and calories

Cuban Cuisine
Nutrition Facts

Food	Serving Size	Calories	Carbs (grams)
À *la vizcaína*	1½ cups	230	28
Arroz frito	¾ cup	225	36
Calabaza	1 cup	304	43
Cocido de garbanzos	1 cup	211	19
Cuban bread	1 slice	76	15
Cuban sandwich	1 sandwich (6 inches)	699	58
Cuban *tortilla*	1 cup	308	15
Flan	1/2 cup	236	39
Fried *tostones*	1 cup	262	39
Fried yuca	6 pieces	340	49
Ropa vieja	1 cup	271	5
Sancocho	1 cup	372	36

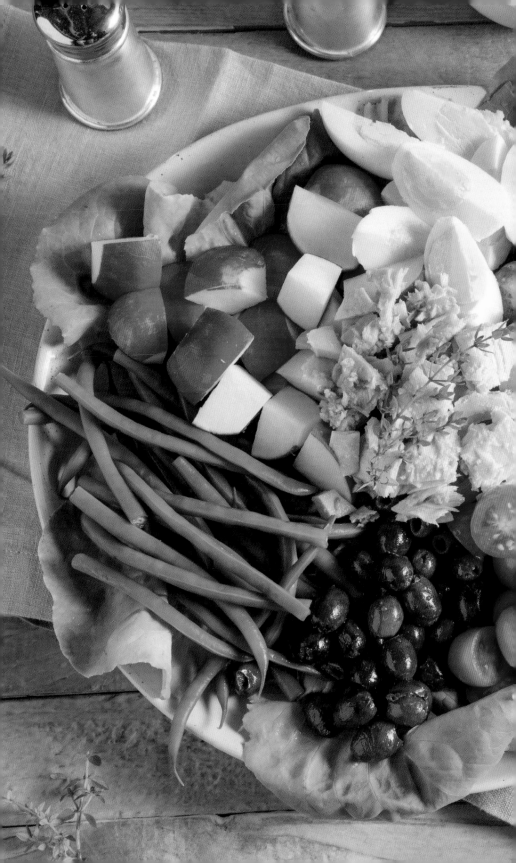

ENJOYING THE FOODS OF

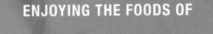

French Cuisine

French cuisine is often thought of as elaborate, but it should not be intimidating. Most dishes, which can fit into any healthy diabetes meal plan, start with a *mirepoix*, a combination of celery, onions, carrots, and garlic. French dishes are often rounded out with healthy herbs like thyme, basil, and parsley.

Strategies for Healthy Eating

Focus on fish and poultry. The French love fish and seafood. Fish is a great option as it is a natural source of omega-3 fatty acids and relatively low in calories. Poultry, a low-fat meat, also plays a notable role in the French diet.

Go for legumes. Naturally low in fat and high in fiber, legumes like beans, peas, and peanuts are a great choice for plant-based protein. In France, lentils, chickpeas, and fava beans are frequently used in soups, baked in casseroles, and served in cold salads.

Enjoy fresh vegetables. Consumed as accompaniments to entrées, by themselves, and in salads, vegetables play a substantial role in the French diet. Try to fill at least half of your plate with vegetables at lunch and dinner.

Avoid creamy sauces and fried foods. Many dishes in French cuisine use rich, creamy sauces that are high in fat. Consider smaller portions of these types of sauces. Tomato-based, broth-based, or vegetable-based sauces are lower in fat and calories.

Eat sweets in moderation. The French are famous for their rich and delicate dessert specialties. In fact, being able to create cakes and fine pastries is considered an art form in France. Foods like croissants— either plain or filled with chocolate—can be high in fat, sugar, and calories. If you choose a frozen treat like a sorbet (which is simply blended fruit and sugar), you'll limit your fat intake. But don't forget that the sorbet's high sugar content can cause a rapid rise in your blood glucose. Limit your serving size to a half cup.

Healthy Pleasures

Bouillabaisse Soup made with a variety of fish and shellfish, including snapper, clams, mussels, scallops, and shrimp, as well as vegetables like potatoes and tomatoes; stewed in a broth seasoned with a variety of herbs, cayenne pepper, and salt

Moules marinière Mussels steamed with white wine, shallots, laurel leaf, and thyme

> **TIP** *This dish is usually served with fried potatoes. To save on fat and calories, consider a salad as your side dish.*

Potage St. Germain Mint-infused pea soup; an excellent source of fiber

Ratatouille Medley of vegetables—eggplant, zucchini, bell peppers, tomatoes, garlic, and onions—individually sautéed, then baked with olive oil, salt, pepper, and a mix of herbs, such as marjoram, fennel, basil or bay leaves, and thyme

Salade niçoise Salad made with tuna, hard-boiled eggs, potatoes, anchovies, tomatoes, olives, lettuce, and other raw vegetables

> **TIP** *While this dish has many health benefits, don't overdo it on the potatoes, which are high in carbohydrates.*

Dishes Reserved for Special Occasions (or Smaller Portions)

Chicken *cordon bleu* Chicken breast wrapped around ham and cheese, then breaded and fried; finished with a drizzle of creamy *hollandaise* sauce made with egg yolk and butter; high in fat and carbohydrates

Crêpes Very thin, unleavened pancakes typically topped with either sweet (when filled with cheese or fruit) or savory (when filled with stuffed meat, poultry, fish, or seafood) sauces; sweet *crêpes* can be high in fat and carbohydrates, and savory *crêpes* can be high in fat and sodium

Filet de boeuf béarnaise Filet of beef covered in *béarnaise* sauce made with clarified butter, egg yolks, vinegar, and herbs; low in carbohydrates but very high in fat and sodium

French onion soup Soup made of onions and beef or chicken stock topped with a browned crust of bread or croutons and grated cheese; a single cup contains a hefty amount of saturated fat and carbohydrates

Pâté de foie gras *Pâté* (spreadable paste) made with fatty goose liver that often includes truffles and added pork fat; made with either milk or heavy cream, which is carbohydrate free but very high in fat

Quiche lorraine Pastry baked with a filling of cream, beaten eggs, and bacon; high in carbohydrates and saturated fat

French Cuisine
Nutrition Facts

Food	Serving Size	Calories	Carbs (grams)
Bouillabaisse	1 cup	90	10
Chicken *cordon bleu*	4 oz	240	15
Crêpe, fruit filled	1 *crêpe* (3 oz)	143	21
Filet de boeuf béarnaise	3 oz beef	156	0
	2 Tbsp sauce	155	1
French onion soup	1 cup	378	42
Hollandaise sauce	2 Tbsp	161	½
Moules marinière	3½ oz	172	7
Oysters, steamed	3½ oz	102	6
Pâté de foie gras	3½ oz	201	7
Potage St. Germain	8¾ oz	120	22
Quiche lorraine	11½ oz	810	59
Ratatouille	1 cup	139	13
Salade niçoise	10 oz	310	8

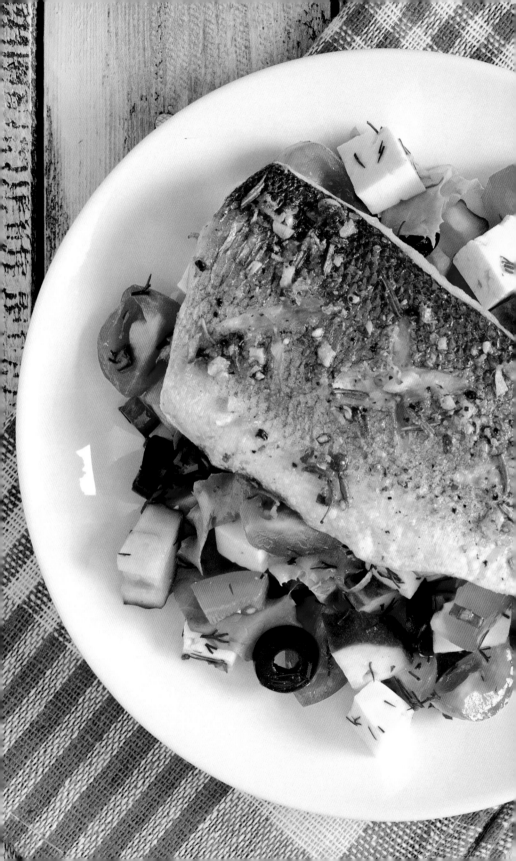

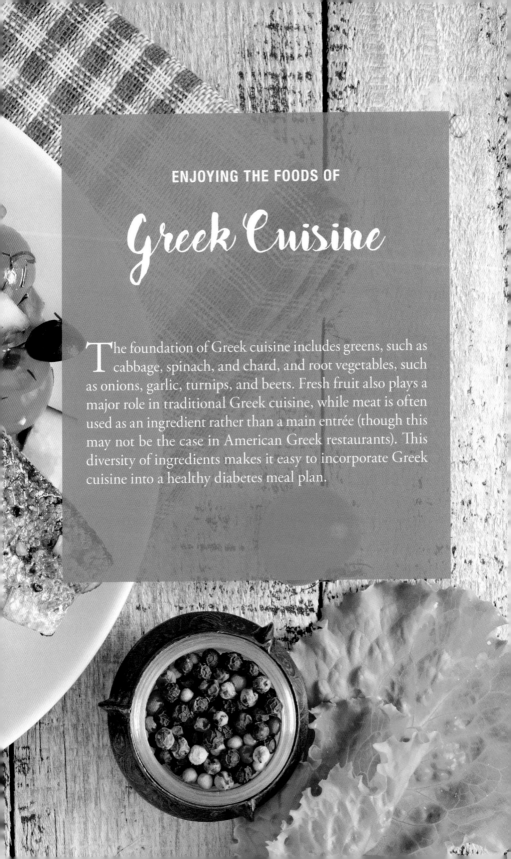

ENJOYING THE FOODS OF

Greek Cuisine

The foundation of Greek cuisine includes greens, such as cabbage, spinach, and chard, and root vegetables, such as onions, garlic, turnips, and beets. Fresh fruit also plays a major role in traditional Greek cuisine, while meat is often used as an ingredient rather than a main entrée (though this may not be the case in American Greek restaurants). This diversity of ingredients makes it easy to incorporate Greek cuisine into a healthy diabetes meal plan.

Strategies for Healthy Eating

Choose kebabs and grilled meat. Grilled fish, chicken, and kebabs are great options that are low in saturated fat. If you have the option, choose this method of preparation in order to limit calorie and fat intake.

Focus on fish and chicken. Lamb, pork, and beef, depending on the cut, may contain substantially more saturated fat (which is known to raise cholesterol) than fish or chicken. If you do choose an alternative meat, opt for lean cuts of pork or lamb.

Control carbohydrates by ordering either pita bread or rice, but not both. Pita bread, rice, and rice pilaf are all high in carbohydrates, and you'll often find that more than one is served at a meal. Keep your blood glucose under control by choosing either pita bread, rice, or rice pilaf at meal times. If you opt for all three, be sure to limit your amount of each in order to stay within your carbohydrate budget.

Remember, beans have carbohydrates too. While beans are a great source of protein (especially when paired with a grain, like brown rice or whole-wheat pita bread), they are not void of carbohydrates. A half cup serving has 15 grams of carbohydrates.

Increase your fiber intake by filling one-half of your plate with vegetables. Fiber helps control blood glucose levels. Remember to find ways to add more vegetables to your meal. Nonstarchy vegetables usually contain only a small amount of carbohydrates per serving.

Choose fresh fruit. Fruits are usually eaten fresh in Greek cuisine, but they are also served dried or as jams and compotes, which means more sugar. Try to stick to fresh fruits whenever possible, and limit your portion to one medium-sized fruit or a half cup serving of fruit salad.

Healthy Pleasures

Dolmas Appetizer consisting of grape leaves typically stuffed with a combination of rice, pine nuts, onions, tomatoes, peppers, zucchini, eggplant, mint, and garlic (and sometimes ground meat)

> **TIP** *Don't forget that the rice in dolmas contributes to your carbohydrate budget.*

Greek salad Salad containing lettuce, tomato, cucumbers, red onions, olives, and feta cheese

> **TIP** *Feta is a very salty cheese, so you'll want to go easy on your portion. One ounce of feta cheese has 260 milligrams of sodium. Select cheeses with fewer than 200 milligrams of sodium per ounce.*

Grilled chicken A chicken breast (or other cut) marinated in olive oil and lemon juice, cooked on a charcoal grill, and served with saffron-infused white rice and seasonal vegetables

> **TIP** *Choose a portion of rice that fits within your carbohydrate budget, or fill no more than a quarter of your plate with it.*

Grilled whole fish Whitefish cooked on a grill and topped with olive oil, lemon juice, oregano, and fresh garlic; often served with risotto and a side of steamed seasonal vegetables

> **TIP** *Risotto is a rice dish that counts toward your carbohydrates for the meal. Choose a portion of risotto that fits within your carbohydrate budget, or skip the risotto and have an extra portion of steamed vegetables.*

Souvlaki Small cubes of lamb, chicken, or pork threaded and roasted on a skewer, either served on the skewer or in a pita sandwich and garnished with *tzatziki* sauce made of Greek yogurt, cucumbers, garlic, salt, olive oil, lemon juice, and a variety of herbs, such as dill, mint, and parsley

> **TIP** *Save on carbohydrate content by ordering souvlaki on a skewer. The calories in tzatziki sauce can add up fast thanks to the olive oil. To control portion size, ask for tzatziki on the side.*

Stuffed cabbage Cabbage leaves stuffed with ground lamb, beef, rice, and onions and topped with tomato sauce

 TIP *Remember that nonstarchy vegetables are low in carbohydrates and usually contain less than 5 grams of carbohydrates per serving. Always try to fill at least half of your plate with vegetables, as the fiber will help balance your blood glucose levels.*

Dishes Reserved for Special Occasions (or Smaller Portions)

Baklava Pastry made of sheets of phyllo dough layered with a walnut, almond, or pistachio filling and then soaked in a syrup flavored with honey, brandy, rose water, or orange-blossom water; very high in total and saturated fat and carbohydrates

Falafel Ground chickpeas seasoned with cumin, coriander, parsley, and cilantro; formed into balls, deep-fried, and often served in a pita pocket with lettuce and hummus; low in carbohydrates but has an abundance of fat; carbohydrate content will increase when served with a pita pocket and hummus

Gyros Sandwich made with slices of ground beef and lamb or chicken; seasoned with herbs and spices, such as chili powder, coriander, paprika, parsley, and oregano, and slowly cooked on a rotisserie; served wrapped in pita bread and topped with onions, tomatoes, and *tzatziki* sauce; Greek-style pita bread is more dense and higher in carbohydrates than American-style pita; also high in sodium

Moussaka Greek version of lasagna, with layers of baked eggplant, meat sauce (which traditionally includes ground meat, olive oil, onions, garlic, oregano, and basil), potatoes, and a white sauce made with butter; high in total and saturated fat

Spanakopita Crisp, oven-baked savory pie consisting of layers of crisp phyllo dough, spinach, feta cheese, and fresh herbs; high in carbohydrates and very high in total and saturated fat; feta cheese contributes a hefty amount of sodium

Greek Cuisine
Nutrition Facts

Food	Serving Size	Calories	Carbs (grams)
Baklava	1 piece (2" x 2" x 1½")	334	29
Dolma	1 roll (2 oz)	91	8
Falafel	1 piece (approx 2¼" diameter)	86	5
Greek salad, without dressing	1 salad (12 oz)	240	15
Grilled chicken	3 oz	156	0
Grilled whole fish, halibut	3 oz	94	0
Gyro (with pita bread, beef, lamb, onions, tomato, and condiments)	1 sandwich (14 oz)	651	72
Moussaka	1 cup	199	11
Souvlaki, chicken	3 skewers (3 oz each)	300	6
Spanakopita	1 cup	334	17
Stuffed cabbage with beef and rice	1 cup	181	14
Tzatziki sauce	2 Tbsp	40	2

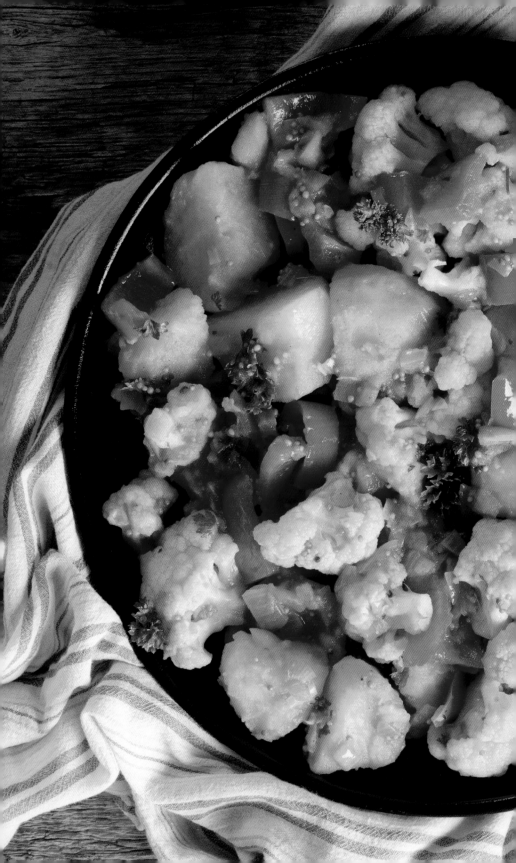

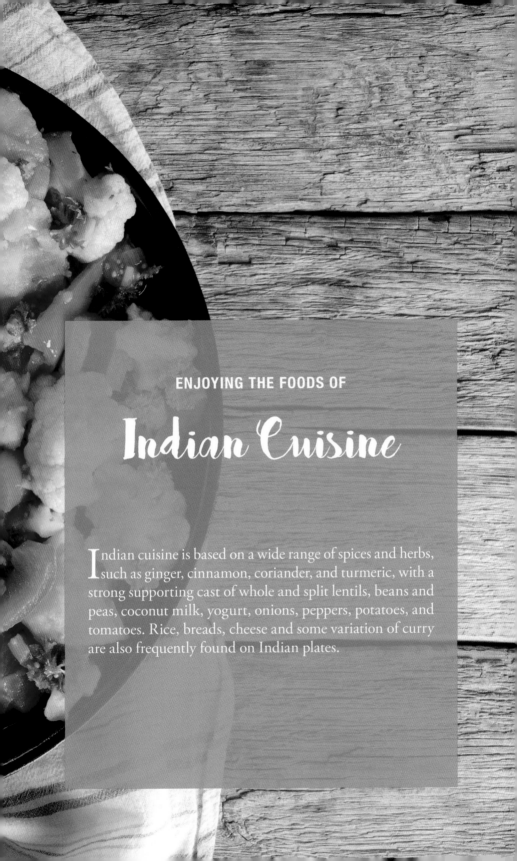

ENJOYING THE FOODS OF

Indian Cuisine

Indian cuisine is based on a wide range of spices and herbs, such as ginger, cinnamon, coriander, and turmeric, with a strong supporting cast of whole and split lentils, beans and peas, coconut milk, yogurt, onions, peppers, potatoes, and tomatoes. Rice, breads, cheese and some variation of curry are also frequently found on Indian plates.

Strategies for Healthy Eating

Remember, beans have carbohydrates too. While beans are a great source of protein (especially when paired with a grain, like brown rice or whole-wheat *naan*), they are not void of carbohydrates. A half cup serving has 15 grams of carbohydrates.

Limit the cheese. Most Indian menus have at least one dish made with cheese. Particularly popular is *paneer*, a fresh cheese made from buffalo milk that resembles cottage cheese. Low in carbohydrates but high in saturated fat (which raises your cholesterol), cheese in Indian dishes should be enjoyed in moderation.

Eat fried foods in moderation. Indian cuisine is full of fried foods, but it's easy to swap fried dishes for healthier options. For example, instead of *papadum,* the paper-thin, crispy, fried *roti* (think Indian tortilla), choose traditional *roti*. Also, you can swap the fried pancake known as *adai* for *idli*, which is similar but steamed.

Load up on vegetables. Many Indians are vegetarians, which means that vegetable-based dishes are not hard to find. Try to devote half of your plate to vegetables whenever possible, as this will help ensure you are getting enough fiber. A favorite recipe along the Indian coast is *bhapa ilish*, a steamed vegetable dish (that sometimes contains fish) seasoned with mustard seed and spices.

Watch the oil. Lots of Indian dishes use copious amounts of vegetable oils—especially peanut oil. While peanut oil may help lower cholesterol and aid in the prevention of heart disease, its calorie content remains the same as other oils, so it should be consumed in moderation. Aim for smaller portions of oil-rich meals when you can.

Healthy Pleasures

Chicken *tikka masala* Bite-sized pieces of chicken marinated in yogurt and seasonings like *garam masala* (a spice mixture that includes black and white peppercorns, cloves, cinnamon, nutmeg, cardamom pods, bay leaf, and cumin), garlic, ginger, cilantro, and turmeric

Chicken *vindaloo* Spicy dish made of chicken marinated in vinegar overnight and then rubbed with sugar, fresh ginger, and toasted spices such as ground peppercorns, mustard seeds, cumin, and coriander; cooked in a sauce made of canola oil, caramelized onions, garlic, ginger, and chilies and served with basmati rice

Dal Pureed lentils or chickpeas; varies in consistency ranging from very thin to pasty.

> **TIP** While lentils are a great source of protein (especially when paired with a grain like semolina, barley, or millet), they are not void of carbohydrates. Try to limit lentils to ta half cup per serving, which is the equivalent of 15 grams of carbohydrates.

Goat *biryani* Tender chunks of goat slow-cooked in rice with herbs and spices, such as chili powder, curry, *garam masala*, ginger, garlic, salt, and saffron; yogurt, *ghee* (clarified butter), and oil are added to provide creaminess

***Tandoori* chicken** Skin-on pieces of chicken marinated in yogurt and seasoned with red chili powder, turmeric, and *tandoori masala*, a spice mix which typically includes *garam masala*, garlic, ginger, onions, and cayenne pepper; baked in an oven

Dishes Reserved for Special Occasions (or Smaller Portions)

Chicken *korma* A curried dish with a thickened nut and yogurt sauce; high in saturated fat, sodium, and carbohydrates

Pakoras Battered and deep-fried vegetables, such as cauliflower, eggplant, or potatoes; high in fat, carbohydrates, and sodium

Saag paneer Spinach or other green leafy vegetables (such as collard or mustard greens) finely chopped and cooked with garlic, ginger, salt, and other Indian spices; thickened with cream or coconut milk and mixed with cubes of fresh *paneer* (cheese); high in total and saturated fat and sodium

Samosas High-carbohydrate and high-fat fried pastries made of flour, butter, salt, and yogurt filled with an assortment of vegetables, such as potatoes, onions, tomatoes, and peas, and seasoned with spices, such as *garam masala*, red pepper, and turmeric; also high in sodium

Indian Cuisine
Nutrition Facts

Food	Serving Size	Calories	Carbs (grams)
Chicken *korma*	2 cups	461	15
Chicken *tikka masala*	4¼ oz	148	7
Chicken *vindaloo*	5 oz	190	7
Dal	1 cup	299	45
Goat *biryani*	1 cup	292	31
Idli	1 small (1¼" diameter)	77	16
Naan	1 oval (3½ oz)	291	50
Pakoras	10 pieces (4 oz)	148	20
Paneer	3 oz	300	3
Roti	1 small (6" diameter, 1 oz)	71	15
Saag paneer	1 cup	320	11
Samosas	1 cup	348	36
Tandoori chicken	3 oz	274	10

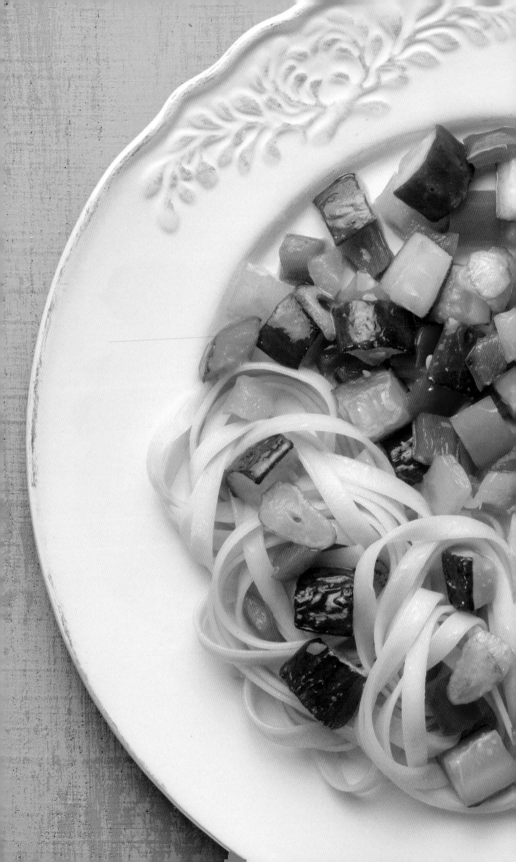

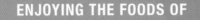

ENJOYING THE FOODS OF

Italian Cuisine

Italian cuisine can be characterized by its simplicity, with many dishes having only four to eight ingredients. Broad differences exist between northern and southern Italian cooking styles; northern fare uses more butter, dairy products, rice, potatoes, and meat than southern fare, which is notable for its use of olive oil, fish, beans, and vegetables, such as artichokes, eggplants, bell peppers, and tomatoes.

The flavors of Italy can be easily incorporated into a healthy meal plan. Limiting the use of rich sauces, choosing vegetable-based dishes laden with fresh herbs and spices, and opting for fresh fruits for desserts will help you enjoy healthy Italian cuisine while managing your diabetes.

Strategies for Healthy Eating

Decide how you want to allocate your carbohydrate budget. Many Italian foods can be high in carbohydrates, so it's helpful to consider your carbohydrate budget in advance of meal planning or decide to divide your carbohydrates between pasta and bread.

Focus on fish and seafood. Many types of fish and seafood are rich in heart healthy omega-3 fatty acids and fit in well as part of a healthy diet. Limit your consumption of pan-fried and deep-fried fish.

Eat pasta and other starches in moderation. Keep an eye on portion size, as carbohydrate content can add up quickly. Order appetizer portions of pasta dishes. Avoid pasta stuffed with meat; instead, opt for plain pasta. Pasta dishes and breads, when eaten along with vegetables and salads, will balance the meal, help you feel satisfied, and improve your blood glucose levels following the meal.

Limit rich sauces. Avoid dishes using the following descriptors: *alfredo, parmigiana, carbonara, saltimbocca,* or creamy. Ask for sauces, grated cheese, and salad dressing to be served on the side.

Healthy Pleasures

Chicken *cacciatore* Chicken cooked in a pan with mushrooms, fresh tomatoes, white wine, and rosemary

Fettuccine *primavera* Boiled fettuccine pasta served with assorted vegetables, such as broccoli, carrots, corn, zucchini, peppers, cauliflower, and peas

Linguine with clam sauce. Boiled linguine pasta topped with a sauce made with chopped clams, clam juice, onions, garlic, olive oil or butter, Parmesan, lemon juice, parsley, and red pepper flakes

TIP *Lighten this dish by substituting broth for the olive oil or butter,and cutting back on Parmesan cheese.*

Pasta *e fagiole* Soup made with pasta, beans, olive oil, and garlic

TIP *Remember, beans are starchy and contain as many carbohydrate as pasta. Be sure to include them in your carbohydrate budget.*

Spaghetti with *bolognese* **sauce** Boiled spaghetti pasta served with a tomato sauce made of sautéed ground pork or beef, olive oil, basil, oregano, and garlic typically topped with grated cheese

Dishes Reserved for Special Occasions (or Smaller Portions)

Cannoli Tube of crisp, fried pastry dough filled with a sweet, creamy mixture of ricotta cheese, sugar, spices, and cocoa powder; may include chocolate chips, dried fruits, or nuts; high in total and saturated fat and carbohydrates

Chicken *parmigiana* Breaded and deep-fried chicken topped with melted mozzarella cheese and marinara sauce; high-sodium, high-fat dish with notable levels of carbohydrates

Fettuccine *alfredo* Boiled fettuccine pasta topped with a white sauce made with cream, butter, nutmeg, and Italian cheese, such as Parmesan or Romano; high in total and saturated fat, carbohydrates, and sodium; opt for fettuccine *primavera* instead to lower fat intake

Lasagne Sometimes spelled "lasagna." Boiled flat noodles layered with a *bolognese* meat sauce and ricotta, mozzarella, and Parmesan cheese; some versions also contain sausage slices; high in total and saturated fat as well as carbohydrates and sodium

Tiramisu Popular coffee-flavored Italian dessert made of ladyfingers dipped in coffee, layered with a whipped mixture of egg yolks, egg whites, sugar, and *mascarpone* cheese, dusted with cocoa powder; the egg yolk and cheese mixture contribute to high saturated fat for the dish

Italian Cuisine
Nutrition Facts

Food	Serving Size	Calories	Carbs (grams)
Cannoli	1 mini (1 oz)	100	12
Chicken *cacciatore* without pasta	3½ oz	184	5
Chicken *parmigiana* without pasta	3½ oz	211	12
Fettuccine *alfredo*	8 oz	581	53
Fettuccine *primavera*	9½ oz	293	34
Lasagne	1 cup (8 oz)	292	31
Linguine with clam sauce	1 cup	354	45
Pasta e *fagiole*	1 cup	228	33
Spaghetti with *bolognese* sauce	11½ oz	310	48
Tiramisu	2½ oz	250	24

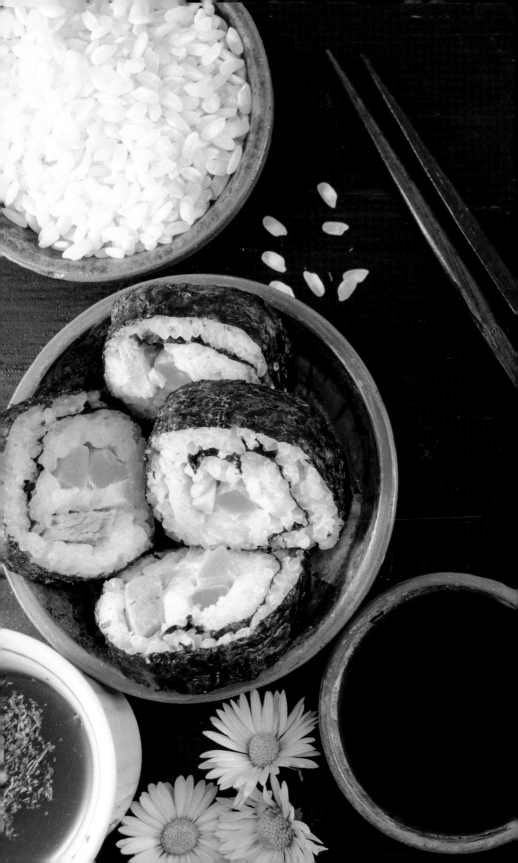

Japanese Cuisine

While starch is often the base of a Japanese meal, generally in the form of rice, this cuisine is all about fresh and seasonal fruits and vegetables that are perfect for a healthy diabetes lifestyle. With the exception of *tempura*, most Japanese dishes use low-fat cooking techniques. However, a potential challenge with this cuisine is soy sauce, which provides much of the flavor and sodium in Japanese food.

Strategies for Healthy Eating

Substitute seafood or chicken for beef. Grilled, baked, or broiled fish, chicken, and shrimp are tasty alternatives to beef dishes, which can be high in saturated fat, depending on the cut. For example, 3 ounces of beef tenderloin has nearly 6 grams of saturated fat, and 3 ounces of baked skinless chicken breast has less than 1 gram of saturated fat.

Ask for sauce and salad dressing on the side. Sometimes, an innocent-looking sauce, such as *teriyaki*, can contain a considerable amount of salt and sugar. Always ask that your sauce and dressing is served on the side so you can control how much goes into your meal. Constraining your portion size of sauces and dressings to 1 tablespoon can greatly reduce the amount of added sodium and sugar in your meal.

Ask that the sauce is made without sugar. If you're lucky, you can ask the chef to change the composition of your sauce entirely. Always check to see if you can get a batch of sauce made with less sugar, which is optimal for blood glucose control. Of course, when preparing your favorite recipes at home, you can use a nonnutritive sweetener instead of sugar or simply reduce the amount of sugar called for in the recipe.

Order brown rice instead of white. Not all restaurants offer brown rice as an option, but many do. Ask your waiter if you can get a side of brown rice instead of white. Remember that a third-cup serving of any kind of rice has 15 grams of carbohydrates.

Avoid high-fat cooking methods such as deep-fried, battered and fried, or breaded and fried. *Tempura*, a popular fried food in Japanese cuisine, is to be indulged in sparingly. Baked, broiled, steamed, and grilled foods are healthier choices.

Healthy Pleasures

Edamame Boiled green soybeans packed with protein and fiber

Miso **soup** A soup containing tofu, fermented soybean paste, and *dashi*, a clear stock made of dried fillets of bonito (a fish) and kelp

TIP Miso *soup is high in salt, so limit the amount you eat. One cup contains over 1,500 milligrams of sodium.*

Ramen Wheat-based noodle served in a broth; can be paired with a variety of toppings, such as sliced pork, green onions, mung beans, or seaweed

TIP *Avoid instant ramen, which is high in sodium.*

Sashimi Thinly sliced raw fish served without rice; a more carbohydrate-friendly choice than *sushi*; accompanied by pickled ginger and *wasabi* (a root vegetable similar to horseradish)

Sushi A combination of raw seafood, vegetables, and sometimes tropical fruit wrapped in seaweed and steamed rice; like *sashimi*, accompanied by pickled ginger and *wasabi* (a root vegetable similar to horseradish)

Dishes Reserved for Special Occasions (or Smaller Portions)

Chicken *teriyaki* Broiled or stir-fried chicken served with a small amount of sliced, sautéed vegetables (typically red peppers and onions) and flavored with a sweet *teriyaki* sauce made of soy sauce, sugar, rice wine, or sake; the sauce boosts the sodium and carbohydrate content

Decadent *sushi* rolls Some rolls contain deep-fried ingredients (such as tempura), mayonnaise (such as spicy tuna rolls), or cream cheese (such as Philadelphia rolls); often high in sodium, fat, and carbohydrates

Salmon *teriyaki* Broiled salmon served with stir-fried asparagus, broccoli, or string beans in a sweet, brown sauce that is high in sodium and carbohydrates

Tempura Shrimp, whitefish, carrots, zucchini, cauliflower, or string beans battered and deep fried; a high-fat, crispy dish

Yaki udo Pan-fried wheat noodles, cabbage, and shiitake mushrooms served in *dashi* stock; high in fat and carbohydrates

Japanese Cuisine
Nutrition Facts

Food	Serving Size	Calories	Carbs (grams)
Edamame (frozen, shelled)	1 cup	188	14
Ginger, pickled	1 Tbsp	30	7
Miso soup	1½ cups	50	6
Ramen soup, mostly noodles	1 cup	156	21
Sashimi	6 pieces (3½ oz)	144	0
Sushi			
California roll	6 pieces (6 oz)	168	36
Tuna roll	6 pieces (6 oz)	174	30
Tempura roll	6 pieces (7 oz)	381	78
Spicy tuna roll	6 pieces (6½ oz)	300	54
Philadelphia roll	6 pieces (5 oz)	345	56
Tempura, vegetable	1 cup	144	12
Teriyaki, chicken, without rice	6 oz	340	14
Teriyaki, salmon, without rice	6 oz	400	8
Wasabi	1 tsp	15	3
Yaki udon	1 cup	287	40

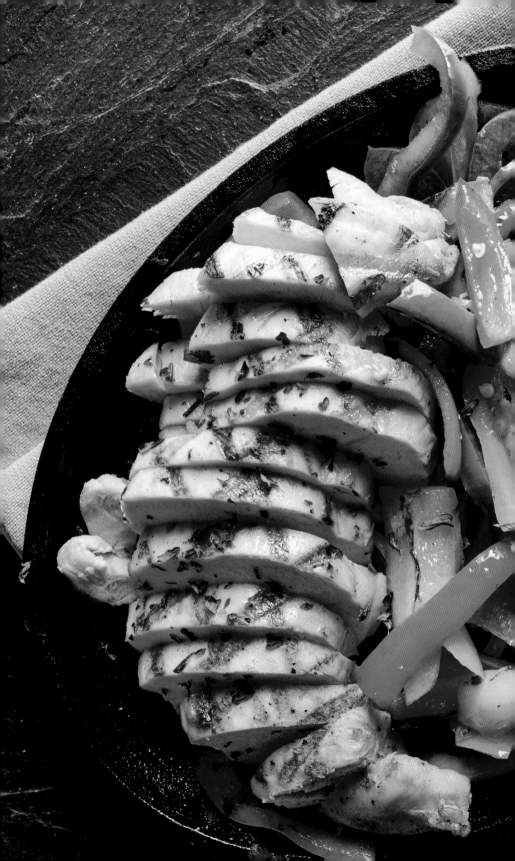

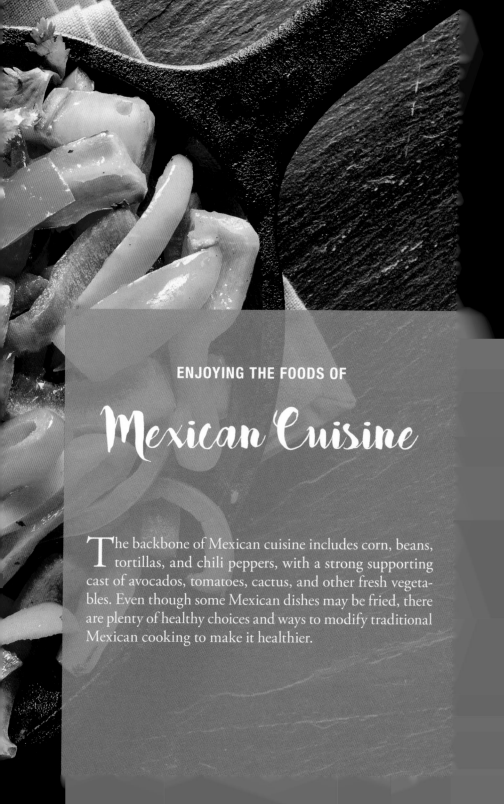

ENJOYING THE FOODS OF

Mexican Cuisine

The backbone of Mexican cuisine includes corn, beans, tortillas, and chili peppers, with a strong supporting cast of avocados, tomatoes, cactus, and other fresh vegetables. Even though some Mexican dishes may be fried, there are plenty of healthy choices and ways to modify traditional Mexican cooking to make it healthier.

Strategies for Healthy Eating

Choose soft tortillas. Frying adds fat and calories, so choose soft tortillas over deep fried whenever possible. For example, choose soft shell *tacos* instead of hard shell (fried) ones, and *burritos* or *enchiladas* instead of deep-fried *chimichangas*. Corn tortillas, known as *arena* in Spanish, have fewer calories and are lower in carbohydrates than flour tortillas. If you choose flour tortillas, look for whole-grain flour tortillas whenever possible.

Beware of chips and cheese. Chips and cheese are a part of many meals in Mexico. Try to limit your portions of both, as they can be high in calories and carbohydrates. Cheese is also high in sodium and saturated fat, so opt for salsa or guacamole instead of cheese when possible.

Go easy on extras. Limit extra calories in Mexican dishes by taking it easy with the add-ons, such as cheese, sour cream, guacamole, and sauces. Replace fatty dressings and sour cream with a tomato-based salsa instead. Your best bets for sauces are red, green, and yogurt sauces.

Consider the preparation method of beans. When making menu selections in restaurants, choose black beans over refried beans. When cooking at home, use canned nonfat refried beans instead of regular refried beans.

Opt for lean meats. Skinless chicken breast is leaner than ground beef, and certain cuts of beef, such as round and sirloin, are leaner than skin-on chicken. Fish and seafood (as long as they aren't fried) are lean options for fillings in *tacos*, *fajitas*, and *burritos*. For example, 3 ounces of beef tenderloin has nearly 6 grams of saturated fat, whereas 3 ounces of baked skinless chicken breast or baked fish has less than 1 gram of saturated fat.

Choose healthy fats. When cooking at home, substitute vegetable oil in recipes that call for salt pork, bacon fat, or lard.

Healthy Pleasures

Burrito Large tortillas stuffed with ground beef, seafood, or shredded chicken (typically seasoned with cumin and oregano), and generally beans, rice, cheese, lettuce, and salsa

TIP *Bean, seafood, or chicken burritos are healthier choices. Reduce carbohydrates by opting for a burrito bowl, which skips the tortilla.*

Enchilada Tortillas stuffed with shredded meat (chicken, beef, or seafood), cheese, beans, onions, and peppers; seasoned with salt, green chilies, oregano and basil; covered with cheese and enchilada sauce (vegetable oil, tomato puree, chili powder, garlic powder, salt, cumin, oregano, and chicken stock); often baked

TIP *Opt for chicken, seafood, or bean enchiladas, and replace some of the cheese topping with vegetables or salsa. Enchiladas are not always baked; they may be fried. When eating away from home, be sure to ask how your enchiladas are prepared to ensure they are diabetes friendly.*

Fajita Grilled chicken, beef, or shrimp served with tortillas and a medley of fresh vegetables (peppers, onions, and garlic) sautéed in vegetable oil

TIP *To make your fajitas more heart healthy, choose chicken breast or shrimp. Limit the number of tortillas to one or two to save on calories and carbohydrates.*

Taco Soft shell tortilla (corn or flour) filled with ground beef, chicken, pulled pork, or seafood and often topped with avocado, lettuce, tomato, and cheese

Quesadilla Flour tortillas filled with cheese, chicken, beef, pork, sausage, or vegetables grilled or pan fried

TIP *Go easy on the cheese in your quesadilla, and choose vegetables or chicken instead of beef, pork, or sausage.*

Arroz a la Mexicana Long-grain rice and vegetables served in a red sauce made of tomatoes, onion, garlic, and chicken broth

> **TIP** *When preparing rice at home, boost your fiber intake by using brown rice or adding extra vegetables.*

Mole poblano Sauce made of a variety of chili peppers, chocolate, nuts, seeds, and spices

Dishes Reserved for Special Occasions (or Smaller Portions)

Atole High-carbohydrate cornmeal-type beverage made with milk or water and sugar

Cajeta Thick, creamy, cinnamon-flavored caramel sauce made with goat's milk; high in carbohydrates and fat

Chimichanga Tortillas filled with beans, meat, or chicken and deep fried; high in sodium, carbohydrates, and fat

Dulce de leche Carbohydrate-rich, thick, and creamy caramel sauce made with cow's milk

Flan Fat- and carbohydrate-rich custard dessert topped with a layer of caramel

Huevos reales Egg-based dairy-free dessert with raisins; high in fat and carbohydrate content

Mexican Cuisine
Nutrition Facts

Food	Serving Size	Calories	Carbs (grams)
Atole	8 oz	209	41
Burrito, bean (fast food)	1 whole (7 oz)	406	62
Cajeta	1 oz	153	33
Chimichanga	5 oz	330	45
Dulce de leche	1 Tbsp	60	11
Enchiladas, chicken, no cheese	6¾ oz	189	21
Fajitas, grilled chicken, no tortillas	8 oz	373	34
Flan	½ cup	236	39
Huevos reales	5 oz	311	46
Arroz a la Mexicana	1 cup	280	51
Mole poblano	¼ cup	78	6
Quesadilla, chicken	1 whole (6⅓ oz)	529	43
Taco, soft, chicken	1 whole (5 oz)	255	27
Tortilla chips	10 chips (⅔ oz)	91	12

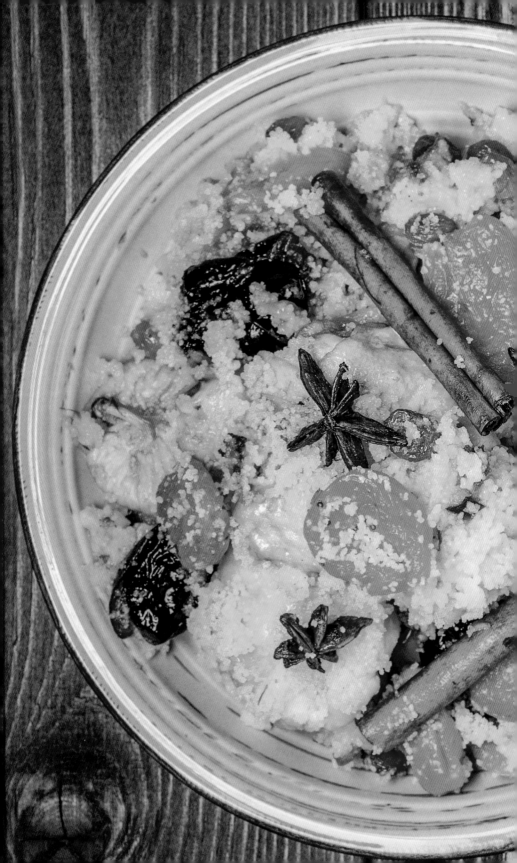

ENJOYING THE FOODS OF

Moroccan Cuisine

Moroccan food is as flavorful as it is healthy. Some of the flavors you can expect to enjoy in this region include coriander, turmeric, ginger powder and cardamom. In fact, one of the most popular dishes in Moroccan cuisine, *tagine*, uses the perfect blend of these spices. Most *tagines* are cooked with vegetables, a grain, and some type of meat or fish. The great news is that like *tagine*, most common Moroccan foods can be part of a healthy diet, even for those who have diabetes or other health issues.

Strategies for Healthy Eating

Focus on fresh fruits and vegetables. You'll find no shortage of fruit and vegetable dishes in Moroccan cuisine. Because they are both high in fiber and low in calories, fruits and vegetables are ideal choices for people with diabetes.

Choose legumes for protein. Legumes are used extensively throughout Moroccan cuisine, and they provide a powerful punch of protein. The combination of protein and fiber in beans will help stabilize your blood glucose levels.

Eat sweets in moderation. While processed sweets are a tasty treat, you should limit your consumption of them, as they are relatively high in calories, simple carbohydrates, and fat.

Opt for complex carbohydrate foods. Choose complex carbohydrate foods, such as bulgur, sweet potatoes, turnips, and potatoes, whenever possible because the fiber in these complex carbohydrates will slow the release of sugar into the bloodstream. When it comes to *couscous*, a type of pasta that is a staple of Moroccan cuisine, choose whole-wheat varieties.

Don't shy away from seafood. Bordered by the Atlantic Ocean and the Mediterranean Sea, Morocco offers a host of delicious fish and seafood dishes that are very healthy options.

Healthy Pleasures

Bissara Soup or dip popular in both Egypt and Morocco made with dried, pureed broad beans; most recipes also include garlic, olive oil, lemon juice, and spices; served in a shallow bowl and topped with cumin, paprika, and olive oil

Couscous Quick-cooking grain made of small steamed balls of semolina usually served with a stew spooned on top

TIP *Opt for whole-wheat couscous whenever possible, as it contains more fiber per serving than regular couscous.*

Harira Popular soup containing *tadouira* (a thickening agent made from water and flour), tomatoes, lentils, chickpeas, onions, rice, eggs, olive oil, herbs, and spices, along with a small amount of meat; can be eaten as an appetizer or light snack; derived from the Arabic word meaning "silky," a reference to the thin consistency of this dish

Loubia Thick tomato and white bean soup containing many spices, garlic, and often carrots; typically served with hot, crusty bread

Moroccan fish *tagine* (*mqualli*) Classic fish, potato, tomato, and pepper dish cooked in a ceramic pot (the pot is also called a *tagine*) or deep skillet over a fire or the stove; typically is served in a sauce made with saffron, ginger, and oil; often includes olives and slices of lemon for additional flavor

Taktouka Cooked salad made with a mixture of tomatoes, green peppers, garlic, and spices served either warm or cold; usually accompanied with crusty bread

Zaalouk Roasted eggplant and tomato salad featuring olive oil, garlic, and herbs; many Moroccan salads are also served pureed as a dip for bread

Dishes Reserved for Special Occasions (or Smaller Portions)

Baklava Pastry made of sheets of phyllo dough layered with walnut, almond, or pistachio filling, soaked in a syrup flavored with honey, brandy, rose water, or orange-blossom water; very high in total and saturated fat and carbohydrates

Ghoriba Starchy shortbread cookie made of sugar, butter, and almonds; okay in small quantities, but large amounts can increase carbohydrate count quickly

Halwa chebakia Pretzel-shaped dough that is deep fried, soaked in honey, and decorated with sesame seeds; packed with sugar

Harsha High-calorie and buttery fried bread made from semolina flour

Kaab el ghzal Sweet pastry filled with almond paste and sprinkled with sugar; can be high in calories

Pastilla Sweet and savory meat pie made by stuffing a thin, flaky pastry shell with poultry or red meat, eggs, and in some cases fried almonds; high in carbohydrates

Moroccan Cuisine
Nutrition Facts

Food	Serving Size	Calories	Carbs (grams)
Baklava	1 piece (2" x 2" x 1½")	334	29
Bissara	1 cup	295	36
Couscous	1 cup	176	36
Fish *tagine* (*mqualli*)	2 cups	358	20
Ghoriba	1 cookie	116	11
Halwa chebakia	1 medium cookie	85	13
Harira	1 cup	218	22
Harsha	3½ ounces (about 1 piece of bread)	384	46
Kaab el ghzal	1 cookie	175	12
Loubia	1 cup	209	12
Chicken *pastilla*	1 piece (about 1½ cups)	590	30
Taktouka	1 cup	220	12
Zaalouk	1 cup	70	15

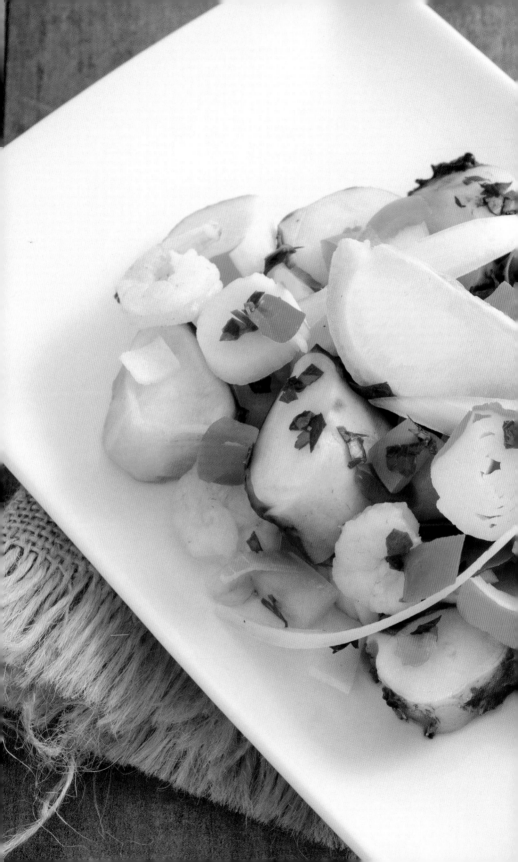

ENJOYING THE FOODS OF

Peruvian Cuisine

Steeped in rich history and heritage, traditional Peruvian cuisine relies on a wealth of indigenous ingredients for its dishes, including potatoes, corn, and beans. Its culture and cuisine include influences from Europe, Africa, and East Asia. From spicy soups and savory stews to seafood-based to rice and bean dishes, the many flavors and cooking methods offer a variety of dining choices that can be as healthy as they are delicious.

Strategies for Healthy Eating

Focus on seafood. Peruvian cuisine is rich in tasty (and heart healthy) seafood dishes. Most of the seafood dishes are low in carbohydrates, and the protein in seafood will help balance your blood glucose levels.

Enjoy fresh fruits and vegetables. Vegetables, such as the cabbage and carrots commonly found in Peruvian dishes, are low in calories, high in fiber, and filled with antioxidants. Try to devote half of your plate to vegetables—especially the green, leafy varieties. While potatoes and yuca are also vegetables, they are very starchy.

Eat sweets and desserts in moderation. Small amounts of Peruvian sweets, such as *mazamorra morada*, can be included in a healthy diet. But remember: Most of the calories in cakes, pies, and tarts come from their carbohydrate and fat content.

Ditch the fried foods. Peruvian cuisine doesn't shy away from fried foods, and many of its main dishes are often paired with fried potatoes or fried yuca as a side. It's best to ask for a serving of vegetables or a side salad instead of a fried option whenever possible, or split the fried potatoes or fried yuca with your dining companions. In general, stick to sautéed, baked, grilled, boiled, or broiled cooking methods whenever possible.

Healthy Pleasures

Aji de gallina Stew of chicken topped with a creamy yellow sauce that contains *aji amarillo* (yellow chilies), milk, pecans, Parmesan cheese, onions, garlic, and spices, as well as bread or crackers; usually served with potatoes and very popular in the winter months

Causa Layered potato salad similar to a casserole that is always served cold, typically as a side dish; traditionally includes layers of potato and avocado, but often also include tuna, meat, tomatoes, or hard-boiled eggs

Ceviche Raw fish marinated in citrus juice, essentially "cooked" in the acid content; typically spiced with red onions and *aji* chilies

Chupe de camarones Chowder of prawns, fish, cream, cumin, tomatoes, potatoes, broad beans, onions, garlic, and spices; usually served with a fried egg

> TIP *If you're making this dish, reduce the amount of cream or substitute low-fat milk to lower the calories and saturated fat.*

Conchitas a la parmesana Simple dish consisting of fresh bay scallops, butter, and Parmesan cheese, typically served on a half-shell; cooked in a double boiler until the cheese has melted but the scallops are only lightly cooked, which helps them remain fresh and soft

> TIP *While this dish is relatively low in carbohydrates, cheese and butter can up the saturated fat. Split this with your dining companions as an appetizer, so you don't overdo it.*

Loma saltado Beef, flame cooked in a wok and smothered with native ingredients, such as *aji* chilies, tomatoes and red onions, to provide a distinctive smoky flavor; one of Peru's most popular meat dishes; often served with fried potatoes

> TIP *Ask for a side of vegetables instead of fried potatoes to boost this dish's fiber and nutrient content.*

Parihuela Spicy soup jam-packed with seafood; usually contains fish heads and bones, fish fillets (such as snapper), mussels, clams, calamari, prawns, scallops, flour, onions, tomatoes, oil, and spices

Pollo a la brasa Roasted chicken marinated in a soy-based sauce flavored with red peppers, garlic, and cumin

Tiradito More delicate version of *ceviche*; contains thinly sliced fish and seafood marinated in a tiger's milk (meaning a citrus-based) sauce and seasoned with chilies, salt, and spices

Dishes Reserved for Special Occasions (or Smaller Portions)

Anticuchos Marinated spiced meat skewers; tends to be high in saturated fat

Mazamorra morada High-calorie and high-carbohydrate Peruvian purple corn rice pudding spiced with cinnamon and cloves

Papa a la huancaína Appetizer of cold lettuce topped with yellow boiled potatoes and a slightly spicy, rich, and creamy cheese sauce called *huancaína* sauce; typically very high in carbohydrates and calories

Papas rellenas Croquettes filled with spicy ground beef stir-fried with onions, tomatoes, garlic, cumin, and paprika; crust is made of hard-boiled eggs, black olives, and mashed potatoes, which raises the calorie and fat content

Sausages and fries Thinly sliced and pan-fried hot dogs or sausages mixed with fried potatoes and topped with sauces; popular Peruvian fast-food option high in carbohydrate and calorie content

Tacu tacu Starchy Peruvian rice and bean patty or pancake that also includes bacon, onions, and spices; usually served with a fried egg; Chefs often make variations that include such ingredients as chilies, asparagus, leeks, mangoes, or avocados

Peruvian Cuisine
Nutrition Facts

Food	Serving Size	Calories	Carbs (grams)
Aji de gallina	1 cup	315	17
Anticuchos	3½ oz	180	2
Causa	2 cups	259	39
Ceviche	½ cup	78	5
Chupe de camarones	1 bowl (about 1½ cups)	719	37
Conchitas a la parmesana	1 shell (1 scallop)	165	1
Loma saltado	1 plate (about 1 cup)	450	42
Mazamorra morada	¾ cup	283	72
Papa a la huancaína	2⅛ cups (2 cups plus 2 Tbsp)	784	137
Papas rellenas	1 cup	513	35
Parihuela	1⅛ cups (1 cup plus 2 Tbsp)	260	8
Pollo a la brasa	¼ of a chicken	510	11
Sausage and fries (does not include sauce)	1 link (3½ oz) about 25 fries	479	90
Tacu tacu	1/3 cup	235	46
Tiradito	1⅛ cups (1 cup plus 2 Tbsp)	285	6

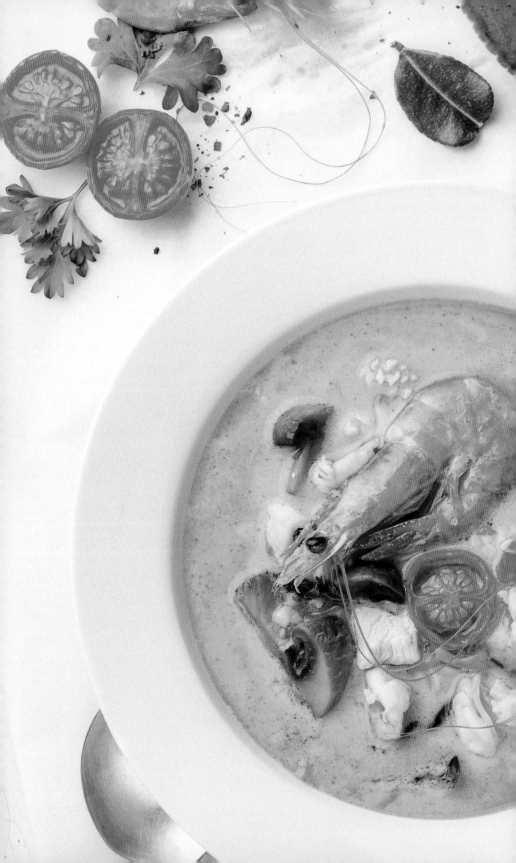

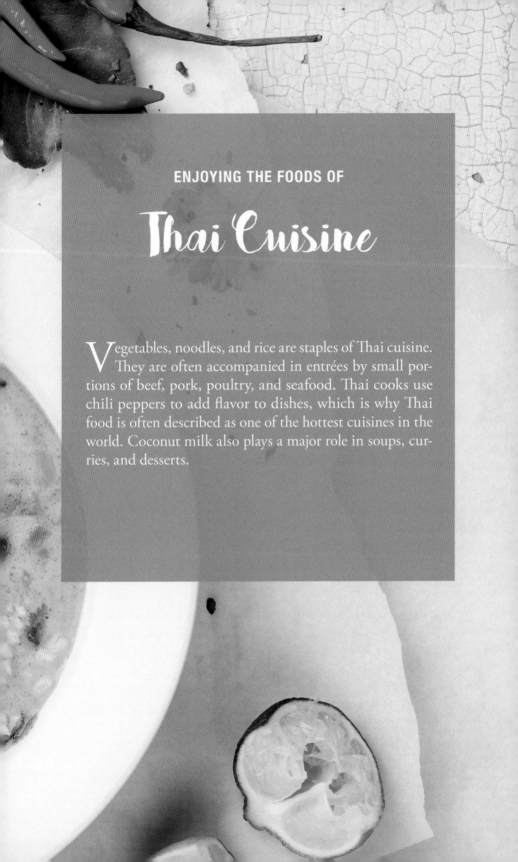

ENJOYING THE FOODS OF

Thai Cuisine

Vegetables, noodles, and rice are staples of Thai cuisine. They are often accompanied in entrées by small portions of beef, pork, poultry, and seafood. Thai cooks use chili peppers to add flavor to dishes, which is why Thai food is often described as one of the hottest cuisines in the world. Coconut milk also plays a major role in soups, curries, and desserts.

Strategies for Healthy Eating

Be aware of fat content. Choose seafood or chicken rather than beef in your Thai dishes. Grilled, baked, or broiled fish and shrimp are tasty and healthy options. Avoid fried duck, which is loaded with saturated fat. Many Thai soups, curries, and desserts are made with coconut milk, which makes them high in fat (unless light or lower fat coconut milk is used). Opt for clear-broth soups, like crystal noodle soup, rather than creamy soups. Peanuts, cashews, and peanut sauces are common additions to many Thai dishes. Opt to leave nuts out of your dishes, and instead of peanut sauce, try a lighter sauce, such as *tamarind* sauce.

Eat rice and noodles in moderation. Portion control is a must when it comes to rice—whether it's white or brown—and noodles. These are high-carbohydrate foods, and overconsumption of them can affect blood glucose levels. Half of your plate should be filled with nonstarchy vegetables, and rice or noodles should be no more than a quarter of your plate. Fill the remaining quarter with a lean protein choice.

Focus on vegetables. Always choose dishes with vegetables in their descriptions, such as vegetable boat, *pad jay* (vegan version of *pad thai*), or vegetable fried rice. When dining out, make sure to ask the server to add extra vegetables to your order, or order steamed vegetables on the side.

Watch out for sodium and sugar. Yellow bean paste, shrimp paste, and fish sauce are high in sodium, and sugar is used in many Thai dishes. When dining out, be sure to specify that no monosodium glutamate (better known as MSG) is used, and be sure to request the sauce on the side so you can control the amount you consume. Many Thai restaurants provide low-sodium soy sauce as an option.

Healthy Pleasures

Chicken and vegetable mini spring rolls Appetizer of chicken, cucumber, carrots, lettuce, and cilantro rolled into rice wrappers

Pad kee mao Flat noodles sautéed in vegetable oil with beef, chicken, or seafood and scrambled eggs, garlic, onions, bell peppers, and carrots, combined with a sauce made of fish sauce, dark soy sauce, rice vinegar, garlic, chilies, onions, and Thai basil

> **TIP** *To reduce the dish's carbohydrate content, consider requesting a smaller portion of noodles and extra vegetables.*

Pad Thai (also *phad Thai* or *phat Thai*) Rice noodles stir-fried with scrambled eggs, vegetables, and beef, chicken, seafood, or tofu; topped with peanuts and a sauce that contains tamarind, fish sauce, shallots, red chili peppers, and sugar

> **TIP** *It's best to ask your server to leave off the peanuts, but if you can't resist, ask for a smaller portion. Don't forget to count the noodles as part of your carbohydrate budget.*

Pad woon sen **with shrimp** Thin glass noodles (made from mung beans or yams) sautéed in vegetable oil with shrimp, scrambled eggs, scallions, baby corn, carrots, and onions; tossed with a mixture of soy sauce, fish sauce, oyster sauce, and garlic

> **TIP** *To reduce sodium intake, ask if your dish can be made with low-sodium soy sauce.*

Spicy Thai-style chicken noodle soup Broth-based soup of seasoned chicken, vegetables, noodles, and chili peppers

Dishes Reserved for Special Occasions (or Smaller Portions)

Basil fried rice Steamed jasmine rice sautéed in vegetable oil with scrambled eggs, onions, bell peppers, garlic, and red chili peppers; tossed with a mixture of oyster sauce, fish sauce, sugar, and Thai basil; high in sodium and carbohydrates

Crispy duck Battered, fried duck basted with soy sauce; high in fat and contains higher amounts of carbohydrates, especially in large portions

Gluay kaeg Banana slices dipped in coconut batter and fried; high in fat and carbohydrates

Red curry with chicken Chicken, bamboo shoots, bell peppers, sugar, and Thai basil simmered in a red curry sauce, which is made with coconut milk and red curry paste (the paste contains garlic, chilies, lemongrass, galangal, cumin, and coriander); coconut milk and sugar boosts the carbohydrate and fat content

Satay Beef, chicken, or pork marinated in coconut milk and curry that is skewered and grilled; served with peanut sauce; can be high in fat content

Thai chicken soup with red curry Soup made with chicken, eggplant, green beans, red curry paste, and coconut milk; high-fat and high-carbohydrate; packs a hefty amount of sodium

Tom ka gai High-fat, coconut milk-based soup containing chicken, mushrooms, and lime juice

Thai Cuisine
Nutrition Facts

Food	Serving Size	Calories	Carbs (grams)
Basil fried rice	¾ cup	180	34
Crispy duck	3½ oz	225	8
Gluay kaeg	1 cup	411	53
Pad kee mao	1 cup	249	34
Pad Thai with seafood	1 cup	290	30
Pad woon sen with shrimp	1 bowl (8 oz)	160	18
Red curry with chicken	1 cup	201	14
Satay, chicken	3 oz	150	5
Spicy Thai-style chicken noodle soup	1 cup	110	17
Spring rolls, vegetable	2 rolls (2 oz)	110	15
Thai chicken soup with red curry	1 cup	200	23
Tom ka gai	1 cup	180	5